Diabetic Smoothie Recipe Book

By

G. Noble

Diabetic Smoothie Recipe Book

By

G. Noble

Published By: Unicorn Publishers
Copyright © 2021 G. Noble.

All rights reserved. No portion of this book may be reproduced in any form without permission from the publisher, except as permitted by U.S. copyright law.

Cover Design By:

S. Pablo

Content Source:

southdenver
medicalnewstoday
healthline
diabeticfoodie
thegestationaldiabetic
kitchennostalgia
&
diabetesstrong

Table of Content

A Diabetic Smoothie Is What It Sounds Like 6

Smoothies: Are They Beneficial To You? 7

Smoothies And Their Beneficial Effects On Diabetes 8

What The Problem Is 9

Remedy 9

Take Care 11

    01. Consume A Variety Of Fats That Are Beneficial To Your Health 12

    02. Include Protein 13

    03. Consume Sufficient Fibre 13

    04. Boost Taste Without Adding Sugar 15

    05. Include Three Carbohydrate Portions 16

    06. Turn It Into A Meal 17

    07. Fruits And Vegetables With A Low Glycemic Index 18

    08. Incorporate Bulk 20

    09. Suggestions For Smoothie Ordering 20

    10. Additional Factors To Consider 21

Advantages of Smoothies 23

Possibilities 24

Ingredients That Are Ideal For Diabetic Smoothies 25

Smoothies For Breakfast That Will Not Elevate Your Blood Sugar 27

The Appropriate Balance 28

- *01. Begin with a liquid. 29*
- *02. Select a Protein 30*
- *03. Include Some Fruits 30*
- *04. Choose A Vegetable 31*
- *05. Choose A Healthy Fat 32*
- *06. Add Flavour And Nutrition Without Sugar 33*
- *07. Make A Meal Of It 34*

The Finest Diabetic-Friendly Smoothie Recipes 35

01. Dragon Fruit Smoothie Bowl 35

02. Smoothie Bowls Made with Peanut Butter and Banana 38

03. Oatmeal Smoothie For Diabetic Breakfast 41

04. Smoothie With Spinach (Low-Carb & Gluten-Free) 42

05. Smoothie With Strawberry Tofu 43

06. Smoothie Of Avocado And Leafy Green Vegetables (Dairy-Free) 46

07. Green Smoothie With Low Carbohydrates 48

08. Low-Carb Mint Watermelon Smoothie 50

09. Blueberry Smoothie Vegan (Low-Carb, High-Protein) 52

10. Smoothie with Chocolate and Avocado (Low Carb, Vegan, Gluten-Free) 55

Take Away 58

Diabetes does not require you to forego all of your favorite foods, but it does require you to make healthier food selections. Consuming a variety of fruits and vegetables, which are high in nutrition but low in calories, is one option.

Certain fruits and vegetables are more effective than others at managing diabetes. Select produce with a low glycemic index and low glycemic load, which means it will not cause a blood sugar spike.

Additionally, it is critical to consume a variety of dairy products that are high in calcium and probiotics to help strengthen your bones and maintain healthy gut bacteria. Low-fat milk, kefir, and Greek yoghurt are all excellent sources of probiotics.

While these foods are necessary components of any diabetes diet, they do not require a fork or even a spoon to be consumed. You can fit a lot of nutrition into a single smoothie and still have a delectable treat. You can enjoy these treats on a regular basis as long as you use healthy ingredients and avoid adding additional sweeteners.

Simply remember to count the fruits you incorporate into your smoothies as part of your daily fruit allowance to avoid carbohydrate overload. Even natural sugars, if consumed in excess, can raise blood sugar levels.

A Diabetic Smoothie Is What It Sounds Like

This collection of diabetic-friendly smoothie recipes features delectable, simple recipes that are low in carbs and sugar-free. Additional points if they are high in protein and fibre.

Because when you consume a nutritious smoothie made with whole foods, you will feel full and energised for hours! There are no blood sugar spikes and no subsequent hunger.

Additionally, they taste quite good. Therefore, whether you're looking for a quick morning snack or an afternoon pick-me-up, this list has something for everyone!

Smoothies: Are They Beneficial To You?

The answer is somewhat complicated... in essence, yes and no. Before we get started with some of my favorite diabetic smoothie recipes, let's discuss why.

Smoothies have grown in popularity as a convenient, healthy breakfast or snack on-the-go. All smoothies, however, are not created equal.

Indeed, many smoothies sold in shops and supermarkets are loaded with sugar and unhealthy ingredients. Certain types are nearly as bad as eating a candy bar!

How do you create nutritious smoothies? The devil is in the details.

Smoothies And Their Beneficial Effects On Diabetes

You may believe smoothies are sugar-laden. While this is true for a large number of store-bought options, you have complete control at home. This is what prompted me to search for recipes for diabetic-friendly, low-sugar smoothies.

What Is The Most Delightful Aspect?

These are not merely delectable confections. These are low-calorie smoothie recipes that will aid in weight loss.

You'll appreciate how quick and easy they are to prepare, particularly on days when you're too busy or lazy to cook. Some days, all you need is a cool, refreshing beverage.

Fruits and vegetables contain nutrients that contribute significantly to balancing your glucose levels while also assisting you in controlling your weight.

It is recommended that you make smoothies from whole fruits and vegetables, not juices, because your body requires a high fibre content, which juices lack.

What The Problem Is

Smoothies are difficult to consume as a diabetic due to their typically unbalanced carbohydrate, protein, and fat content. Additionally, carbs in liquid form enter our system much faster than carbs in solid form. That's already two strikes against you, and all you want is a delectable treat that won't cause your blood sugar to spike. What about on-the-go breakfast shakers? Fasting glucose is already challenging, and you cannot risk shocking your system with a large amount of sugar (even if they are naturally occurring sugars) and experiencing an abnormally high spike, throwing your glucose out of whack for the remainder of the day! That brings the total to three! ...and you could easily be on your way out.

Remedy

A homemade smoothie is the best smoothie for a diabetic. Powdered and frozen smoothie packets, Jamba Juice, Smoothie King, and other 'instant' smoothies either contain added sugars or contain an excessive amount of naturally occurring sugars that mimic the effect of table sugar. By creating your own smoothies from whole foods, you have complete control over the amount of sugar and other ingredients, resulting in a more balanced macronutrient ratio.

Protein powders are not necessary, though they are beneficial and some are quite good. (I adore the Atkins vanilla flavour and almost all of the Shakeology flavours, but chocolate is by far my favourite.) To achieve a balanced smoothie, incorporate high-protein natural foods such as Greek yoghurt, nut butters, and so on.

Smoothie making is an art, which means it is subjective. As a diabetic, you can still enjoy your favorite flavours, but you must prioritise a balanced macronutrient ratio over flavour. To assist you, you should be familiar with the four necessary components of a smoothie: bases, flavourings, sweeteners, and liquids; additives are optional. Download this diabetic smoothie recipe PDF to see which ingredients fit into each category.

This page will be updated frequently with new diabetic-friendly smoothie recipes. The almond berry breakfast smoothie is extremely popular right now, as is the vanilla cake batter shake. My personal favourite is the pina colada smoothie. Listed below are additional smoothie recipes.

Take Care

Avoid gimmicks such as "smoothies for diabetes reversal." Consider this: diabetes did not develop overnight or through the consumption of a single food throughout your life; consequently, there is NO smoothie recipe or single food that will magically reverse diabetes for you, even if you consume it daily for the remainder of your life. This is also true for pregnant women.

Additionally, fruit smoothies are an option, but it makes sense to use low-sugar fruits. Utilize this interactive glycemic index chart to determine the healthiest fruits to incorporate into your smoothies.

Smoothies appear to be a healthy option, and they can be an excellent source of fibre and other nutrients found in fruits and vegetables. However, the wrong type of smoothie can be detrimental to diabetics, particularly when dining out.

Smoothies are an excellent way to incorporate superfoods like spinach and green leaves into your diet. Other ingredients, on the other hand, may be high in fat and sugar, posing a risk of blood sugar spikes and weight gain.

Following a few simple guidelines can help a diabetic person enjoy smoothies while minimising adverse effects.

Continue reading to learn how to make a nutritious smoothie and about the benefits and risks associated with including smoothies in a diabetes diet.

01. Consume A Variety Of Fats That Are Beneficial To Your Health

Certain types of fats are beneficial to diabetic patients. Fats are necessary for the body, and they can assist in slowing the rate at which sugar enters the bloodstream and leaving the individual satisfied.

Include the following healthy fat sources in your morning smoothie:

- Almond Or Peanut Butter
- Avocado
- Chia Seeds
- Raw Pecans
- Raw Walnuts

However, too much fat can result in weight gain, thus it is critical to maintain a healthy balance of fats.

02. Include Protein

Similar to fat, protein provides several health advantages that are critical for everyone, but notably for diabetics.

Protein-rich foods can inhibit meal absorption, which slows the rate at which sugar reaches the system.

Animal or vegetable protein sources are acceptable. Including protein-rich components in a smoothie can have a number of health advantages.

Protein sources for smoothies include the following:

- Plain, Unsweetened Greek Yoghurt
- Hemp And Other Seeds
- Almonds
- Pea Protein
- Whey Protein.

03. Consume Sufficient Fibre

Fiber is available in two forms: soluble and insoluble.
- Soluble fibre is more difficult for the body to digest. This implies that it takes longer for the energy to be released, lowering the likelihood of a glucose surge.

- Insoluble fibre improves digestive health and decreases food absorption in the gastrointestinal system.
- Fiber can help a person feel fuller for extended periods of time.

These things can assist a diabetic individual by lowering their chances of experiencing:

- A blood sugar increase
- Cholesterol accumulation;
- Weight increase as a result of overeating owing to a lack of fullness.

In these methods, fibre can help reduce the risk of developing different issues associated with diabetes and high blood sugar, as well as improve general health.

The following items with a high fibre content may work well in a smoothie:

- The Majority Of Fruits, Including Raspberries, Oranges, Nectarines, Peaches, And Blueberries
- Veggies, such as spinach and kale;
- Nuts; and
- Chia Seeds.

04. Boost Taste Without Adding Sugar

Numerous foods already include sugar, and some have hidden sugars. Sugar is frequently added to processed or prepared foods.

Bear in mind the following while selecting ingredients:
- Certain canned fruits are stored in sugar-sweetened syrups
- Honey And Maple Syrup Are Also Sugars;
- Ripe fruits have more sugar than less ripe fruits;
- Milk includes lactose, another sugar; and
- Almond, soy, and other milk replacements may have additional sugar.

These could be appropriate in moderation.

Other options to add taste include the following:
- A dash of spice, such as cinnamon, nutmeg, ginger, or turmeric;
- Fruit, which offers natural sugar and fibre;
- Nuts; and
- Oats, which may provide a creamy texture.
- Dates and dried fruit in moderation
- Fresh herbs such as mint, basil, or coriander
- Cocoa powder, unsweetened
- Unsweetened coffee
- unsweetened peanut butter

It is preferable to sweeten smoothies with natural components rather than artificial sweeteners.

05. Include Three Carbohydrate Portions

When preparing a smoothie, a person with diabetes must be aware of the carbohydrate content.

In general, patients with diabetes should aim for smoothies with 45 grams or less carbs. It's a good idea to include at least three different carbohydrate types.

Several examples of 15 gm carbohydrate servings that are frequently included to smoothies include the following:

- 1 banana, tiny
- 1 cup of melon
- 3/4 cup blueberries
- 1 cup plain yoghurt
- ½ cup granola

Greens, spinach, or other dark leafy vegetables can be added to the smoothie. These have less carbohydrates per serving and provide nutritious value.

Measuring the amount of carbs in the smoothie with measuring cups, spoons, and the diabetic exchange list is a smart way to do it.

A doctor will advise on the amount of carbohydrate that an individual should consume each day and at each meal — this amount will vary according to an individual's height, weight, activity level, and medicines.

06. Turn It Into A Meal

While a smoothie may appear to be a drink, it can have the same amount of carbohydrates and calories as a complete meal.

Calculate the carbohydrate and calorie content of the smoothie and use it to replace a meal or as a light snack.

If the temptation to have a full breakfast or lunch persists, go for sparkling water, unsweetened tea or coffee as a beverage.

07. Fruits And Vegetables With A Low Glycemic Index

The glycemic index (GI) of a food item indicates how rapidly it raises blood sugar.

In general, a food with a lower GI score indicates that the body will absorb sugar more slowly than a food with a higher GI score. This indicates that foods with a low glycemic index have a lower risk of causing a blood sugar increase.

Water has the lowest GI score of 0, while glucose has the highest at 103.

All fruits and vegetables have a distinct GI score due to their differing sugar and fibre content.

The following are some examples of items that a person could use in a smoothie, along with their GI rating:

Low Glycemic Index Foods (55 Or Less):
- Oranges
- Banana
- Dates
- Plain yogurt
- Mango
- Carrots (boiled)
- Porridge, rolled oats
- Some types of milk, including soy milk.

Foods With A GI Of 56–69:
- Pineapple
- Boiling pumpkin
- Sweet potato

Meals With A High Glycemic Index (70 Or Greater)
- Quick oat porridge
- Watermelon
- Rice milk.

However, just because a product has a low GI score does not imply it may be added to a smoothie in any quantity.

When preparing smoothies, it's also important to keep in mind the following:

• Even if a fruit has a low GI score, the carbohydrate content must still be considered.
• As a fruit ripens, its GI score increases.
• Juicing, blending, or cooking improves the score. Orange juice, for example, has a higher GI than an orange whole, because the sugar is absorbed more quickly by the body.

08. Incorporate Bulk

While a smoothie may appear to be a meal, it is actually a meal replacement. If a person still need a meal to feel full, they should decrease their smoothie intake.

According to one source, 150 milliliters (ml) of smoothie per day should suffice.

Alternatively, you could add water to dilute the solid ingredients.

- Adding water to dilute the solid ingredients
- Increasing the volume of ice.

09. Suggestions For Smoothie Ordering

When ordering a smoothie away from home, inquire about the ingredients and the staff's ability to produce one without added sugar. If they are unable to do so, it is best to choose another beverage.

Certain establishments will prepare the smoothie while the customer waits, allowing them to specify specific ingredients.

10. Additional Factors To Consider

Diabetes patients may also develop additional conditions and complications, such as hypertension, obesity, celiac disease, and lactose intolerance.

These additional conditions may restrict the types of ingredients that can be included in a smoothie.

a. Intolerance To Lactose

Individuals who are lactose intolerant should avoid adding dairy milk or dairy milk byproducts, such as yoghurt, to a smoothie.

Almond milk or soy milk are both acceptable substitutes for dairy milk in the majority of smoothie recipes.

Individuals should choose unsweetened milk alternatives or verify the sugar content of a product prior to purchasing and using it, as some milk alternatives may contain a significant amount of sugar.

b. Gluten Intolerance

Celiac disease is more prevalent in people with type 1 diabetes than in the general population, according to studies.

Celiac disease sufferers must avoid foods containing gluten, a protein found in wheat, rye, and barley.

Whey protein is one component that, depending on the brand, may include gluten. While whey is naturally gluten-free, some producers add gluten-containing additives to their products.

Always read the label before purchasing whey products or experimenting with alternative plant-based proteins.

c. Insufficiency

Individuals who are overweight or obese will need to keep a close eye on their calorie intake. Increasing your intake of plant foods and fibre can assist.

In general, a smoothie that is suitable for someone with diabetes is likely to be acceptable for someone trying to lose weight.

c. Hypertension And Hypercholesterolemia

Individuals with high blood pressure and cholesterol should consume foods that are high in fibre and low in fat, such as:

- Beets
- Nuts and seeds
- Leaves that are green
- Fruits
- Skim milk.

Individuals with hypertension should also avoid meals that have additional salt.

Advantages of Smoothies

Smoothies can constitute a complete meal, including sufficient protein, carbs, fibre, and fat to satisfy an individual for an extended period of time.

Smoothies made with fruits, vegetables, nuts, and seeds may be an excellent source of vitamins, minerals, and other essential elements. Each of these nutrients has the potential to boost an individual's overall health.

Proper nutrition may help a person lower his or her cholesterol, lose weight, develop muscle, support a healthy neural and circulatory systems, and increase energy levels.

Possibilities

When ordering or making a smoothie, it's essential to remember that, despite its appearance as a drink, a smoothie can contain at least as many carbs and calories as a meal. Individuals should avoid consuming a full meal in addition to their smoothie.

Additionally, while smoothie components may contain fibre, mixing food breaks down fibre, making it simpler to digest.

When fruits, vegetables, and other high-fiber foods are consumed in a smoothie rather than whole and unprocessed, they will be less fulfilling and more likely to cause a blood sugar increase.

Individuals should not drink all of their fruit and vegetables in smoothies, but should aim to consume the majority of their meals in whole form.

Ingredients That Are Ideal For Diabetic Smoothies

It's necessary to keep in mind that your smoothie is just as healthy or bad as the components you choose.

There are components that have been shown to help manage blood sugar levels, and smoothies are an excellent way to guarantee you receive them every day!

The American Diabetes Association has compiled a list of the 10 items that every diabetic should consume in order to boost their diet's effectiveness.

These foods have a low glycemic index (GI) and are high in nutrients that are typically lacking in the standard western diet, including calcium, potassium, fibre, magnesium, and vitamins A (as carotenoids), C, and E.

Among the ADA's suggested superfoods, the following are our favourites for diabetic smoothies:

• **Dark Green Leafy Vegetables (spinach, collards, kale)** - due to their low calorie and carbohydrate content, they're a great superfood to use into smoothies.

- **Citrus Fruit (grapefruit, oranges, lemons)** - either freshly squeezed juice or sliced into cubes for an extra dose of soluble fibre. A juicer-blender combination appliance might be advantageous in this case.

- **Sweet Potatoes** - they not only contribute vitamin A and fibre to smoothies, but also a creamy texture and sweetness!

- **Berries** - whatever variety you pick, berries will provide antioxidants, vitamins, and fibre to your smoothies while also adding colour and flavour.

- **Nuts and seeds** – contain beneficial lipids and magnesium. Either add nut butters to your smoothies to increase smoothness, or grind flaxseed to improve the omega-3 fatty acid content.

- **Fat-free Milk and Yogurt** - If you are not a vegetarian, this is the basic liquid for your smoothies.

Smoothies For Breakfast That Will Not Elevate Your Blood Sugar

Smoothies for breakfast can be an excellent way to start the day. Smoothies are an excellent source of protein, fiber, healthy fats, and other nutrients found in fruits and superfoods such as spinach and leafy greens. They cram a lot of nutrition into a small travel cup and can taste more like dessert than a healthy snack or meal.

However, smoothies are not without their drawbacks. If you make a morning smoothie at home or order the incorrect blend at your favourite juice bar, your refreshing beverage can spike your blood sugar and then crash, leaving you queasy and exhausted rather than satisfied.

Even if a smoothie is loaded with healthy ingredients, it can spike blood sugar levels if portions are too large or the smoothie is not made with the proper blend or ratios of ingredients.

When blood sugar levels rapidly rise, the insulin rushes to remove excess sugar from the blood and into the cells, resulting in a blood sugar crash. This can leave you exhausted and hungry, rather than satiated and energized.

If you have diabetes and spike your blood sugar with a smoothie or any other food or beverage, your cells may not respond as well to insulin, causing your blood sugar to remain elevated for an extended period of time. This can result in headaches, fatigue, an increase in thirst, blurred vision, and difficulty concentrating.

Regardless of whether you have diabetes or not, you should limit yourself to a small, 8- to 12-ounce smoothie to avoid blood sugar spikes. This portion contains approximately 175–450 calories, making it an ideal snack or light meal.

The Appropriate Balance

Just as a healthy snack or meal should contain a balance of carbs, protein, and fat, so should a healthy smoothie. This balance is critical for avoiding dangerous blood sugar swings. While there is no 'ideal' ratio of ingredients, a serving of protein, one serving of fruit, a tablespoon or two of healthy fat, and a serving or two of vegetables is a good starting point.

Bear in mind that sweetened yogurts, sweetened non-dairy milk, and juice all contain added sugars. When combined with the fresh fruit that is typically included in smoothies, this amount of sugar is far too high. Even though the sugar in fruit is "natural," not "added," consuming all of that sugar at once without any protein or fat will result in a significant blood sugar spike.

01. Begin with a liquid.

Several low-carb liquid bases for smoothies include the following:

- Drinking water
- Unsweetened almond, hemp, or other plant milk containing approximately 1 gram of carbohydrates per cup
- Unsweetened soy milk is another option, containing only 3–5 gram of sugar per cup.
- On the other hand, cow's milk contains approximately 12 gram of carbohydrates (lactose sugar) per cup. That is not to say that you should abstain from using cow's milk. Simply add less fruit to your blender than you normally would to keep total sugars low and blood sugar spikes at bay.

02. Select a Protein

Protein is critical for slowing down digestion and promoting feelings of fullness and satiation. Smoothies with a high protein content can slow food absorption, which slows the rate at which sugar enters the bloodstream. It's also critical for maintaining muscle mass, which aids in blood sugar regulation.

- Unsweetened Greek yoghurt
- Cottage cheese
- Silken tofu
- Vegan, rice, pea, or whey protein powder

03. Include Some Fruits

Breakfast is an excellent time to incorporate a fruit serving. Simply ensure that it is a single serving. Too many smoothie recipes contain two to five servings of fruit, which is an excessive amount of sugar to absorb at once.

• A serving contains 3/4 – 1 cup berries, a small banana or 1/2 large bananas, 1 orange or 1/2 grapefruit, and 1/2 cup mango or pineapple.

• Smoothies with frozen fruit have a wonderful texture.

04. Choose A Vegetable

Are you a spinach or kale purist? Instead, sip them. A handful or two of leafy greens are high in antioxidants, potassium, and vitamin K, and contain very little sugar. They blend easily into smoothies without significantly altering the flavor, even if they do give your shake a slight green tint. Some veggie ideas:

- 1-2 handfuls dark leafy greens such as spinach, kale, or Swiss chard
- 1/2 cup cooked pumpkin or sweet potato
- 1-2 small beets and beet greens
- ½ – 1 cup celery or cucumber
- A serving of powdered greens supplement

Fruits and vegetables also contain fibre which is essential to good health. Fiber can be soluble or insoluble. Soluble fibre is more difficult for the body to digest. This implies that it takes longer for the energy to be released, lowering the likelihood of a glucose surge.

Insoluble fibre boosts digestive health and reduces the absorption of other foods in the gastrointestinal tract, which also helps to prevent blood sugar spikes.

Additionally, fibre can help you feel fuller for longer periods of time and can help prevent weight gain as a result of overeating due to a lack of fullness. buildup of cholesterol in the blood.

05. Choose A Healthy Fat

There are many sources of healthful fats that can be used in smoothies, such as avocado and chia seeds. Fats are necessary for the body because they aid in the absorption of fat-soluble vitamins A, D, E, and K found in plants and fruits. Fats can also help slow down the speed at which sugar enters the blood and leave you feeling satisfied. However, too much fat can result in weight gain, therefore it is critical to maintain a healthy balance of fat - around 2 tablespoons is ideal.

Several healthy fat sources to include in a morning smoothie include the following:

- Almond or peanut butter
- Chia, flax or hemp seeds
- Avocado
- Cashews, pecans, walnuts or almonds.

06. Add Flavour And Nutrition Without Sugar

Herbs and spices are nutrient powerhouses. Other ways to add flavour to your smoothie without adding any sugar include:

- A pinch of spice, such as cinnamon, nutmeg, ginger, or turmeric
- Herbs in their natural state, such as mint, basil, or coriander
- . Extracts such as vanilla, almond, peppermint, or others, but not syrups
- Unsweetened cocoa powder, or cacao nibs
- Black coffee.

07. Make A Meal Of It

While a smoothie may appear to be a drink, it can have the same amount of carbohydrates and calories as a complete meal.

Calculate the carbohydrate and calorie content of the smoothie and use it to replace a meal or as a light snack.

If the temptation to have a full breakfast or lunch persists, go for sparkling water, unsweetened tea or coffee as a beverage.

Enjoy!

The Finest Diabetic-Friendly Smoothie Recipes

After exhaustive research I found several extremely fantastic recipes, and also created and tried my own ideas for diabetes friendly smoothies, so here they are.

In several of the dishes you'll find I choose for berries instead of other fruits like melons. This is because berries are reported to contain lower quantity of carbs per serving. This is good for diabetics since it keeps your glucose levels regulated.

It's not to imply that you can't consume other fruits. Absolutely not. Use additional fruits of your choosing but in a restricted quantity.

Feel free to tweak an ingredient or two. Use what you have.

01. Dragon Fruit Smoothie Bowl

Dragon fruit (also known as Pitaya) is a gorgeous fruit that comes in red or white hues. While its remarkable look is what earns it fame, its flavour is what keeps people coming back for more.

The dragon fruit is native to Central American but is now cultivated all over the world. It has a somewhat sweet, delicate taste that some equate to a pear combined with a kiwi. The dragon fruit goes wonderfully with other tropical fruits such as pineapple, mango, and guava.

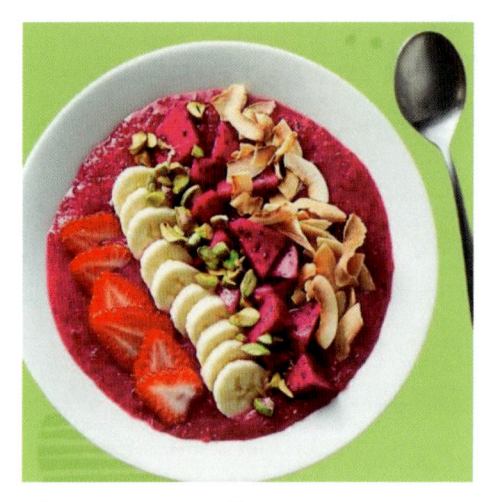

This wild fruit also carries some significant nutrition, featuring an incredible quantity of prebiotic fibre and antioxidants. Dragon fruit may even help increase fasting blood glucose (sugar) levels! A few studies have demonstrated that dragon fruit eating helps lower fasting blood glucose (sugar) in persons with pre-diabetes and type 2 diabetes. Though the effects were more pronounced in persons with pre-diabetes.

Fresh dragon fruit is typically difficult to locate but most grocery shops stock frozen dragon fruit. For this dish, I used a frozen combo of dragon fruit, mangoes, strawberries, and peaches but feel free to be creative and mix in other fruit!

Pro-tips:

- **Add sweetness if required!** I think the fruit was enough to sweeten the bowl, but if you wish you may add a sweetener to taste.

- **Toppings:** Get inventive! I prefer adding a bit of a crunch, so almonds were ideal! Any nuts, chia seeds, flax seeds, or granola would also be a fantastic addition.

- **Put the spinach into the blender first,** this will make mixing the smoothie a bit simpler!
- If you want a drinking smoothie - add some liquid. You can go for your favourite milk or add a juice like pomegranate.

- **Need extra protein?** Add with your favourite protein powder or collagen peptides!

INGREDIENTS:

- .Approximately 3/4 cup frozen fruit
- 1 cup spinach
- 1/2 cup Greek yoghurt
- 1/2 Avocado.

How To Cook Dragon Fruit Smoothie Bowl

1. Add items to blender or food processor.
2. Blend on high until smooth. As required, pause and scrape the edges with a spoon or spatula to incorporate all ingredients.
3. Enjoy!

02. Smoothie Bowls Made with Peanut Butter and Banana

When frozen bananas, soymilk, cocoa powder, chia seeds, and peanut butter are blended together, a creamy, healthy, and delightful smoothie bowl with an astonishing 10 grams of protein and 7 grams of fibre is created.

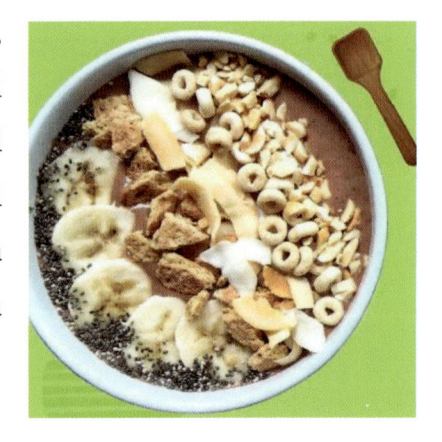

Smoothie bowls come in a variety of hues and tastes (purple, green, orange, yellow, chocolate brown), but their consistency is usually the same: thicker than a drinking smoothie but thinner than pudding. They're supposed to be eaten with a spoon, and the topping possibilities are infinite - nuts, fruit, seeds, coconut, crushed Graham crackers, and whole grain cereal, to name a few!

Equipment Required For Making A Smoothie Bowl: Blender, Bowls, And Spoons.

Blender Ingredients - Use less liquid than a standard smoothie; add thickening ingredients; and include a decent amount of protein and healthy fat. (You require fat in your diet in order to absorb the beneficial elements found in fruits and vegetables.)

- Liquids: 100% fruit or vegetable juices, milk, soy milk, almond milk, or coconut milk.
- Frozen banana, mango, pineapple, strawberries, peaches, raspberries, baby spinach, kale, cucumber, wild blueberries, pumpkin puree, and roasted beets.
- Healthy fats: peanut butter, nut butters, avocado, whole milk or yoghurt with 2% fat, and coconut oil.
- Stabilizers: chia seeds, greek yoghurt, and banana

- Milk, yoghurt, almonds, peanut butter, nut butters, cottage cheese, and protein powder are all good sources of protein.

Ingredients for the Topping

Whole grain cereal, nuts, chia seeds, hemp seeds, sunflower seeds, pumpkin seeds, shredded coconut, coconut chips, fresh fruit, dried fruit, and crumbled graham crackers.

Ingredients

- 1 cup plain or vanilla soymilk
- 2 frozen bananas
- 3 tablespoons peanut butter
- 2 teaspoons chocolate powder
- 1 tablespoon chia seeds
- ¼ teaspoon pure vanilla extract.

Guidance

1. In a blender, combine the soymilk, bananas, peanut butter, chocolate powder, chia seeds, and vanilla.

2. Spoon into separate bowls and decorate with desired toppings.

03. Oatmeal Smoothie For Diabetic Breakfast

This quick and satisfying smoothie is an excellent way to start the day with oats, a blood sugar balancing item. It makes it easier to maintain a healthy blood sugar level throughout the day.

Both oats and flaxseed are high in fibre and also include a variety of vitamins and minerals. Additionally, oatmeal is a cholesterol-free, sodium-free, and fat-free food.

Ingredients

- 1 cup uncooked oats, pounded in a spice or coffee grinder or food processor
- 2 frozen bananas, chopped into small bits beforehand
- 3 cup skim milk
- 2 tbsp powdered flaxseed
- Sugar alternative (optional).

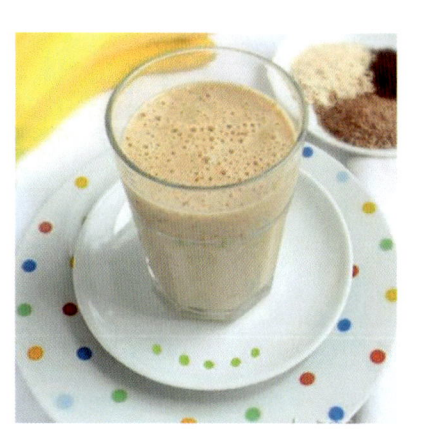

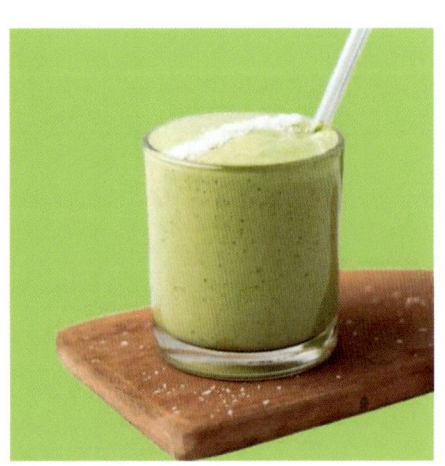

Guidance:

1. In a blender, immersion blender, or food processor, combine all ingredients.

2. Fill a glass halfway with Oatmeal Breakfast Smoothie and serve!

04. Smoothie With Spinach (Low-Carb & Gluten-Free)

This creamy spinach smoothie is enhanced with nut butter, yoghurt, and avocado. It's an excellent way to get your morning dose of leafy greens!

Ingredients:

- 2 tbsp. nut butter
- 12/ cup yoghurt, plain Greek
- 1/2 pitted avocados
- 1/4 cup milk (or almond milk)
- 1 tsp vanilla extract
- 2 cup spinach, fresh
- a few sweetener drops (to taste)
- ice 1 cup

Guidance

1. In a blender, combine everything except the ice.
2. Puree the mixture until completely smooth.
3. Pulse in the ice until most of it is smashed.
4. Puree the contents in a blender until it is smooth and creamy.

Notes

This spinach smoothie recipe yields two servings.

Remaining portions should be refrigerated in an airtight container and consumed within a day or two.

05. Smoothie With Strawberry Tofu

This strawberry tofu smoothie is an absolute must-try! Tofu, almond butter, and almond milk combine to provide the ideal creamy foundation, while strawberries and vanilla essence give a delicious flavour. Lemon juice adds the appropriate amount of acidity to the dish.

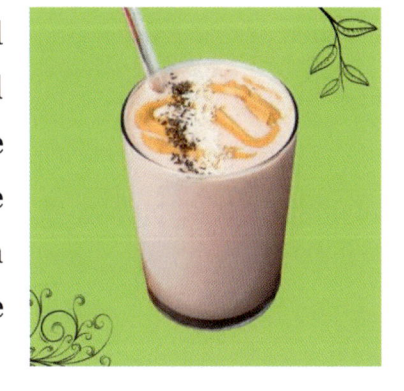

Additionally, this delectable meal has around 16 grams of protein, 18.5 grams of healthy fats, and 5 grams of fibre, making it a nutrient-dense smoothie that you can feel good about sipping.

Enjoy it as an energising breakfast or as a delectable afternoon treat!

Ingredients

- 12 ounces tofu
- 1 cup sliced strawberries
- 1 cup almond milk
- 2 tablespoons almond butter
- 1 teaspoon lemon juice
- 1 teaspoon vanilla extract
- 1/2 cup ice cubes
- 3-5 drops liquid Stevia

Make A Strawberry Tofu Smoothie

Once the strawberries are sliced and the remaining ingredients are prepared, this smoothie comes together quickly!

Step 1: Combine all ingredients except the ice cubes in a blender. Until smooth, blend.

Step 2: Fill the blender halfway with ice cubes and process until perfectly smooth.

Step 3: Serve immediately with chosen toppings.

Creating a smoothie with toppings

This smoothie is wonderful straight from the blender, but you can also top it with your favourite toppings!

After all, who doesn't appreciate a delectable smoothie?

If I'm not pressed for time, I like to top my smoothie with coconut flakes, chia seeds, and a dab of almond butter. Strawberry and almond butter tastes complement each other beautifully, and I adore the crunch provided by the seeds and coconut flakes!

Interested in further suggestions? With sugar-free chocolate chips, there is no such thing as a mistake! Alternatively, for an added crunch, cut some nuts of your choosing and toast them briefly in a skillet.

Decorate your smoothie as you like! Simply remember to calculate the nutritional value of any toppings.

06. Smoothie Of Avocado And Leafy Green Vegetables (Dairy-Free)

Avocado smoothies with leafy greens are an excellent way to boost your intake of healthy fats. Additionally, it's quite simple to prepare — simply combine all ingredients in a blender!

Ingredients

- 2 cups baby spinach
- 1 cup baby kale
- 2 mint sprigs
- 1 avocado (peeled and seed removed)
- 1 tablespoon freshly squeezed lemon juice
- 2 cups water
- 1/2 cup ice cubes

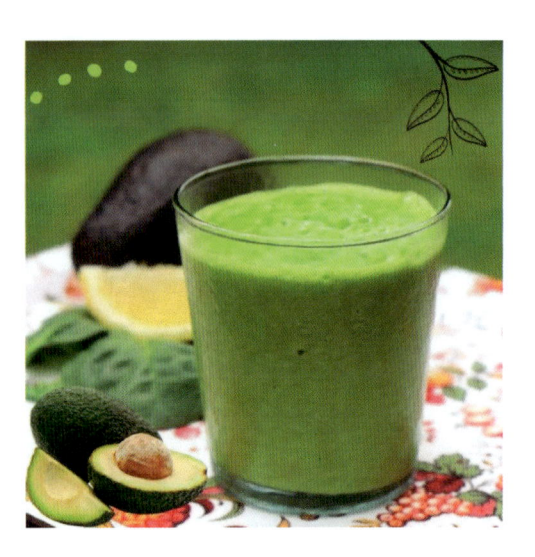

How to make Avocado smoothie recipe with leafy vegetables

Step 1: To begin, fill a high-powered blender halfway with spinach, kale, mint, avocado, lemon juice, and water. Ice cubes should be added at the very end.

Step 2: Blend the ingredients at a high speed until smooth.

Distribute evenly between two glasses and serve immediately!

If you want to add some sweetness, you may add a few drops of Stevia or a drizzle of honey, but I recommend starting with the smoothie. You may discover that you prefer it without the addition of any additional sweetness.

Making The Ideal Green Smoothie: A Few Tips

Make sure your avocado is fully ripe for the best texture. This will result in a smooth, delicious smoothie. If your avocado is overly firm, you may wind up with a thick smoothie that is unappealing.

Additionally, I recommend preparing the entire dish, even if you're only feeding one. Otherwise, your blender's volume may be insufficient to get a smooth texture.

Simply store the remainder in the refrigerator for tomorrow's breakfast or snack!

You might avoid measuring the greens to save time. A cup of greens is equivalent to a couple of handfuls, so grab whatever you like and add it! Additionally, there is no need to remove the stems because the blender will do so for you.

Additionally, you may substitute any greens of your choosing (or happen to have on hand). I've experimented with various mixes of spinach, romaine, and kale and they've all been delicious.

07. Green Smoothie With Low Carbohydrates

This low-carb green smoothie is loaded with protein and beneficial fats! It's very creamy because to the almond butter and avocado, and spinach adds nutrition.

Ingredients

- 1 tablespoon almond butter
- 1/4 cup protein powder (i used isopure vanilla)
- A few drops stevia sweetness
- 1 cup unsweetened almond milk
- 2 cups spinach
- 1 teaspoon vanilla extract
- 12 cup frozen avocado
- 1 cup ice cubes

How To Prepare A Green Smoothie

To make this beautiful smoothie, all you need are seven ingredients, ice cubes, and a blender.

Step 1: Combine all ingredients except the ice cubes in a blender.

Blend until smooth in the second step.

Step 3: Fill the blender halfway with ice cubes and whirl until perfectly smooth.

This concludes the discussion! I serve mine in a glass cup and garnish with shredded coconut and flax seeds.

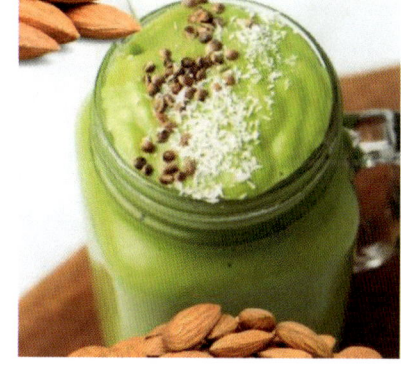

This Smoothie May Be Customised.

You may create this smoothie in a variety of different ways, depending on your interests and preferences.

Are you a lover of almond butter but aren't a huge lover of the flavour? Substitute a different nut or seed butter for this one! Because it contributes to the smoothie's texture, I would not advocate leaving it out totally.

Likewise, you may replace any other milk of your choice for the almond milk. Simply keep in mind that substituting ordinary dairy milk will result in an increase in carbohydrates.

Additionally, you may substitute whatever leafy greens you choose. Although I like spinach in this smoothie, kale, Swiss chard, or even beet greens would work just as well.

Feel free to be inventive and adapt this recipe to your personal preferences for flavour and convenience!

08. Low-Carb Mint Watermelon Smoothie

When the weather is hot, I enjoy having a fast smoothie to chill off.

However, you know what I despise? All of the sugar, fillers, and artificial components found in smoothies purchased from a shop or supermarket.

As a result, I like to make simple smoothies at home, such as this low-carb watermelon smoothie with mint and lime juice! The taste combination is quite refreshing, and this drink comes together in less than five minutes.

If you're in the need for something refreshing or just don't know what to do with leftover watermelon, this dish is a must-try. It just could become a new summer favourite!

Ingredients

- 2 cups diced and cooled watermelon
- 1 lime (juiced)
- 5 drops stevia liquid (or to taste)
- 1/ cup soy milk
- 5-10 mint leaves, fresh (to taste)
- 3 cups ice

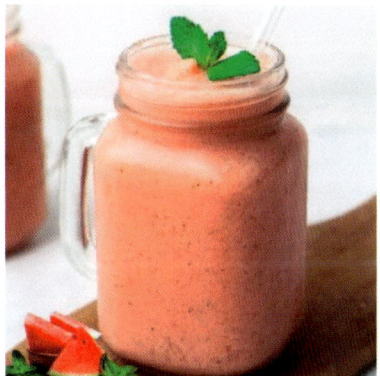

How To Prepare A Low-Carb Watermelon And Mint Smoothie

This very simple smoothie comes together in just four quick steps.

Step 1: In a blender, combine the watermelon, lime juice, stevia, soy milk, and mint.

Step 2: Puree the mixture until absolutely smooth.
Add the ice in the third step.

Step 4: Pulse until smooth, then serve immediately.

Is Watermelon Beneficial To Diabetics?

Watermelon is a refreshing fruit that may be had in moderation as part of a balanced snack or meal.

For instance, this dish calls for 1/2 cup watermelon per serving. Watermelon has around 5.5 grams of carbs, 0.3 grams of fibre, and 4.5 grams of sugar in that quantity.

While this fruit does not have the lowest carbohydrate or sugar content, dishes like smoothies allow you to reduce the serving size while still enjoying the flavour.

09. Blueberry Smoothie Vegan (Low-Carb, High-Protein)

After tasting this homemade, high-protein, vegan blueberry smoothie, you'll never want to purchase another pricey pre-made smoothie again!

This smoothie is so delectable that it has quickly become one of my favourites. I enjoy the thick, creamy texture and the fact that I'm receiving an antioxidant boost. And with only five (clean!) ingredients, I'm guessing it's also more healthier than the majority of pre-made smoothies.

Making this delectable smoothie couldn't be simpler. Simply add all of the ingredients and mix!

This vegan-friendly low-carb smoothie is a nutritious powerhouse, including over 15 grams of protein per cup. As soon as you take a taste, you'll wonder how something so decadent and creamy can be so healthy!

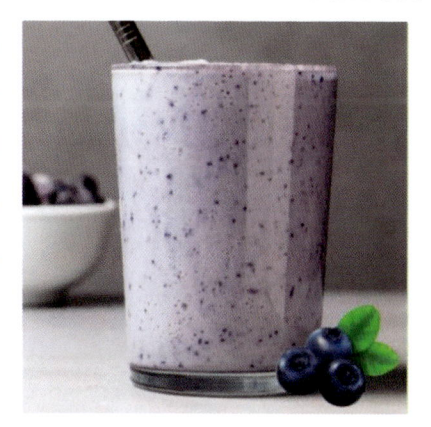

Ingredients

- 14 oz canned unsweetened coconut milk
- 1/2 cup unsweetened almond milk
- 1/2 cup fresh or frozen blueberries
- 4 tbsp pea protein powder
- 1/2 tsp vanilla essence

How To Make A Blueberry Vegan Smoothie

Smoothie recipes are quite simple to prepare. And this dish calls for only five ingredients!

Step 1: In a high-speed blender, combine the blueberries, almond milk, pea protein powder, and vanilla.

Step 2: Gradually add the coconut milk until the smoothie reaches the required consistency.

Step 3: Blend on high speed until all ingredients are well combined and the smoothie is a light purple colour.

All that remains is for you to take a straw and enjoy!

10. Smoothie with Chocolate and Avocado (Low Carb, Vegan, Gluten-Free)

This simple Chocolate Avocado Smoothie with coconut milk is rich, creamy, and packed with a nutritious, delectable mix of ingredients! Additionally, it is low carb, gluten-free, and vegan.

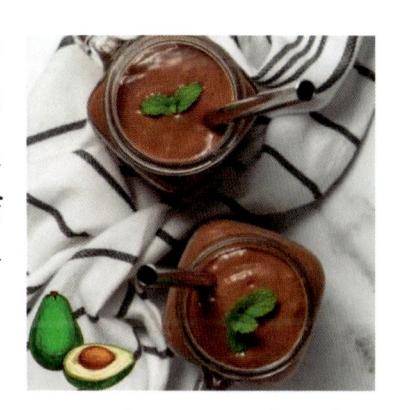

This simple chocolate avocado smoothie is a decadent, creamy delight that will please even the most discerning sweet tooth!

The key is in the avocado's compatibility with cocoa powder. This ingredient transforms the smoothie into a sumptuous delight that is extremely smooth and pleasant!

And when the coconut milk is added for additional creaminess, you get the most lovely texture you can imagine... for less than 80 calories per serving!

That is correct. This delicacy has the appearance of a full day's calories, but owing to the correct combination of ingredients, it is actually rather light and healthful.

Additionally, there are just five primary components required, plus water, salt, and optional mint for decoration. What could be better than healthy, delicious, and incredibly simple to prepare?

Whether you make this smoothie as a post-workout snack, a quick breakfast, or even a dessert, you will be amazed that something so delectable and rich can be low-carb and healthy!

Ingredients

- 1/2 ripe avocado
- 3 tablespoons cocoa powder
- 1 cup full-fat coconut milk
- 1/2 cup water
- 1 teaspoon lime juice
- pinch mineral salt
- 6-7 drops liquid Stevia
- Fresh mint

To Prepare A Chocolate Avocado Smoothie, Follow These Steps.

Preparing the ingredients and blending this delectable dessert takes less than 5 minutes.

Step 1: In a blender, combine all of the ingredients.

Step 2: Using a high-speed blender, blend until smooth and creamy. Add additional liquid Stevia to taste if desired.

Step 3: If preferred, garnish with fresh mint and serve.

It doesn't get much more straightforward than that. Because I generally always have these ingredients on hand, this smoothie is my go-to anytime I'm in the need for something refreshing and chocolaty!

You'll understand why after you try it.

Smoothie Variations

One of the things I love about smoothies is how customizable they are. You may change the ingredients to suit your taste or just what you have on hand!

In my smoothies, I choose liquid Stevia, but any low-carb sweetener would work in this recipe. Please feel free to utilise whatever method works best for you!

Any unsweetened plant or nut milk may be substituted for the coconut milk. If you're not vegan, you may easily substitute a couple tablespoons of yoghurt.

You may also substitute 1/2 a banana for the avocado if you don't have a ripe avocado.

One of my most important advice for this dish is to refrigerate the avocado, coconut milk, and 1/2 cup water ahead of time. The chilly components impart an additional creamy texture to the smoothie. It's very pleasant on a hot summer day!

Take Away

Smoothies may be a healthful and delicious way to start the day or to provide a fruit or vegetable snack in between meals. However, a diabetic should examine the ingredients to ensure there is no added sugar.

It is preferable to create smoothies at home in order to guarantee that they contain nutritious components.

Printed in Great Britain
by Amazon